Exercise
and
Prostate Health

Exercise
and
Prostate Health

Best Practices and Benefits

Victor Asher

Other Books by Victor Asher

Simple Exercise for Osteoporosis

Achieving & Maintaining a Healthy Life

The Inevitable Journey of Grief

Understanding the Quality & Benefits of a Revitalizing Sleep

A Step – By – Step Guide for Dads

Optimizing Life with Osteoarthritis

Unveiling The Hidden Benefits Of Walking And Hiking

Relationship's Hurricanes

Eating For Health

Cook well Eat well and live well

The Enigmatic African Grey Parrot

Understanding & Taming the Fiery Nature of Anger

How to Achieve Financial Stability in Today's World

Coping with Adolescence

Alternative and Complementary Therapies for Rheumatoid Arthritis

The Path to Success

Life Changing Quotes on Pages

Imaginative Tales to Dream Away

Beyond The Throne

60 Mind-loving Stories for Seniors

Dedication

This book is dedicated to God for His grace and wisdom, to my family, to my beautiful readers who will find this book relevant to them, and to everyone who has loved, supported, and encouraged me along the way. I would not be in the position I am in today without your unshakable faith in me. I dedicate this book to all my readers' especially those who have prostate issues as this will sincerely be of importance to you all.

Table of Contents

Acknowledgement

I want to sincerely thank God for providing the means and insight that guided me during the writing of this book. I cannot forget my family members, whose encouragement and support have given me bravery and motivation throughout the process.

Thank you to my editor and publisher for their crucial advice and help in bringing this project to its successful conclusion. I would like to express my gratitude to everyone who so kindly contributed their time and knowledge to this project and added their wisdom. I want to express my gratitude to my friends as well, I appreciate all of your steadfast love and support throughout the journey.

I like to thank atlanticurologyclinics.com, pcfa.org.au and medika.life for your amazing images, you all are wonderful.

Finally, I extend my thanks to each and every one of you for purchasing and reading my work. I am thankful it met your needs and added to your knowledge. I sincerely value each and every one of you and think you're all fantastic.

Introduction

Maintaining optimal prostate health is a vital aspect of overall well-being for men. While factors like age, genetics, and lifestyle choices can influence prostate health, incorporating regular exercise into one's routine has been shown to have numerous benefits. Exercise not only promotes cardiovascular fitness, muscular strength, and flexibility, but it also plays a significant role in supporting prostate health and reducing the risk of various prostate conditions.

In this book, we will explore the best practices and benefits of exercise specifically related to prostate health. We will delve into the connection between exercise and the prostate, examining how physical activity can contribute to the prevention and management of common prostate conditions such as benign prostatic hyperplasia (BPH), prostatitis, and prostate cancer. By understanding the positive impact exercise can have on the prostate, individuals can make informed choices to prioritize their well-being and adopt a proactive approach to prostate health.

Through this comprehensive guide, we will provide valuable insights into suitable exercise modalities, recommended frequencies and intensities, and additional lifestyle factors that can further support prostate health. Whether you are looking to reduce the risk of prostate conditions, enhance urinary function, or complement existing treatment plans, the information presented here will serve as a roadmap for incorporating exercise into your life in a safe and effective manner.

By adopting the best practices outlined in this book and embracing an active lifestyle, men can take proactive steps towards maintaining optimal prostate health and improving their overall quality of life. So let's explore the power of exercise in promoting prostate health and unlock the benefits that physical activity can offer.

Chapter One

Understanding Prostate Health

A. Overview of the Prostate Gland

The prostate gland is an important part of the male reproductive system. It is a small, walnut-sized gland located just below the bladder and in front of the rectum. The prostate gland plays a crucial role in the production and transportation of semen.

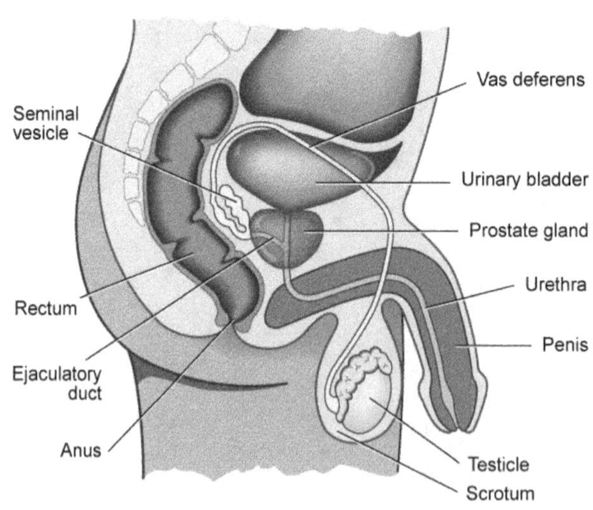

The prostate gland is a muscular and glandular organ that surrounds the urethra, the tube responsible for carrying urine from the bladder out of the body. It consists of three main zones: the peripheral zone, central zone, and transitional zone. The peripheral zone is the largest and most significant in terms of prostate cancer development.

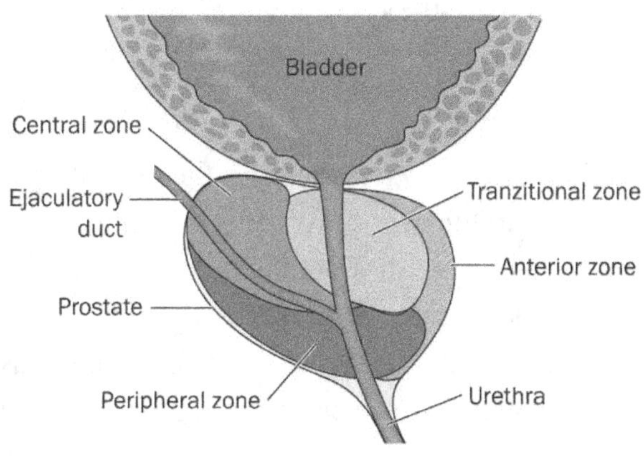

Functions of the Prostate Gland

In the male reproductive system, the prostate gland, which is found slightly below the bladder, serves a number of crucial roles.

These tasks consist of:

1. Secretory Function

The prostate gland is responsible for producing a milky, alkaline fluid that constitutes a major part of semen. This prostatic fluid contains enzymes, proteins, and nutrients that provide nourishment and support to the sperm. It also enhances sperm motility and prolongs their lifespan within the female reproductive tract.

2. Prostate-Specific Antigen (PSA):

The prostate gland produces a protein called prostate-specific antigen (PSA). PSA is primarily used as a screening marker for prostate-related conditions, including prostate cancer. Elevated levels of PSA in the blood may indicate the presence of an issue, such as infection, inflammation, benign prostatic hyperplasia (BPH), or prostate cancer.

3. Role in Ejaculation

During ejaculation, the smooth muscles of the prostate gland contract rhythmically, aiding in the propulsion of semen into the urethra. This muscular action, along with contractions of other reproductive structures, helps expel semen from the body during sexual activity. The prostate's contractions contribute to the forceful release of semen and facilitate the movement of sperm through the reproductive tract for fertilization.

4. Influences Urinary Function

The location of the prostate gland around the urethra can affect urinary function. As the prostate gland enlarges with age, it may constrict the urethra, leading to a condition called benign prostatic hyperplasia (BPH). BPH can cause urinary symptoms like frequent urination, weak urine flow, difficulty starting or stopping urination, and the sensation of incomplete bladder emptying.

5. Sexual Function

The health of the prostate gland can influence sexual function in men. Conditions like prostatitis (inflammation of the prostate) can cause pain and discomfort during sexual activity. Additionally, treatments for prostate conditions, such as surgery or radiation therapy for prostate cancer, may impact erectile function and ejaculation.

It's important to note that any concerns or symptoms related to the prostate gland should be discussed with a healthcare professional. They can provide appropriate guidance, diagnosis, and treatment options based on an individual's specific situation.

B. Common Prostate Conditions

The prostate gland (a walnut-sized gland located just below the bladder in men), is an important part of the male reproductive system. It surrounds the urethra, the tube that carries urine from the bladder out of the body, and produces a fluid that mixes with sperm to create semen. However, the prostate is prone to various medical conditions that can affect its structure and function.

The various medical conditions include:

1. Benign Prostatic Hyperplasia (BPH)

BPH is a non-cancerous enlargement of the prostate gland. As men age, the prostate tends to grow, leading to compression of the urethra and causing urinary symptoms. Symptoms of BPH include frequent urination, weak urine flow, difficulty starting and stopping urination, nocturia (waking up at night to urinate), and urinary retention.

2. Prostatitis

Prostatitis refers to inflammation or infection of the prostate gland. It can be caused by bacteria, viruses, or other factors. Prostatitis can present with symptoms such as pain or discomfort in the pelvic area, frequent and urgent urination, pain during urination or ejaculation, and flu-like symptoms. There are different types of prostatitis, including acute bacterial prostatitis, chronic bacterial prostatitis, chronic prostatitis/chronic pelvic pain syndrome (CPPS), and asymptomatic inflammatory prostatitis.

3. Prostate Cancer

Prostate cancer is a malignant tumor that develops in the cells of the prostate gland. It is one of the most common types of cancer in men. Prostate cancer often grows slowly and may not cause symptoms in its early stages. As it progresses, symptoms may include difficulty urinating, blood in the urine or semen, erectile dysfunction, pain in the back, hips, or pelvis, and unexplained weight loss. Regular screening with prostate-specific antigen (PSA) blood tests and digital rectal exams (DRE) can help detect prostate cancer early.

4. Prostate Stones

Prostate stones are small, calcified structures that can form in the prostate gland. They are usually composed of calcium and other minerals. Prostate stones are relatively common in older men and may be associated with chronic prostatitis. They can cause symptoms such as pain in the pelvic area, difficulty urinating, and recurrent urinary tract infections.

5. Prostate Abscess

A prostate abscess is a collection of pus within the prostate gland. It is typically caused by a bacterial infection and can occur as a complication of acute bacterial prostatitis. Symptoms may include severe pain in the pelvis, fever, chills, difficulty urinating, and blood in the urine. Prompt medical attention and treatment with antibiotics and drainage are necessary to treat a prostate abscess.

6. Prostatic Intraepithelial Neoplasia (PIN)

PIN refers to the presence of abnormal cells in the prostate gland that are considered pre-cancerous. It is often detected during prostate biopsies performed for other reasons. High-grade PIN is associated with an increased risk of developing prostate cancer, although not all cases progress to cancer.

7. Prostate Infections

Prostate infections can occur due to bacterial, viral, or fungal infections. They can be acute or chronic and may result from urinary tract infections, sexually transmitted infections, or other sources of infection. Symptoms include pain or discomfort in the pelvic area, fever, chills, urinary symptoms, and sometimes blood in the urine.

8. Prostate Biopsy Complications

A prostate biopsy is a procedure in which small tissue samples are taken from the prostate gland to check for the presence of cancer or other conditions. While generally safe, it can have potential complications such as bleeding, infection, pain, and discomfort in the rectal area or during urination.

9. Prostate Nodules

Prostate nodules are small, abnormal growths or lumps within the prostate gland. They may be benign or cancerous. Nodules can sometimes be felt during a digital rectal exam (DRE) or detected through imaging tests. Further evaluation, such as a biopsy, is often needed to determine the nature of the nodules.

10. Prostate Atrophy

Prostate atrophy refers to the shrinking or loss of prostate gland tissue. It is most commonly associated with aging and hormonal changes. Although prostate atrophy is generally benign and does not cause significant symptoms, it can sometimes lead to urinary problems or be mistaken for other conditions.

11. Prostate Fibrosis

Prostate fibrosis involves the formation of excess fibrous tissue within the prostate gland. It can be a result of inflammation, injury, or other factors. Fibrosis may cause urinary symptoms similar to BPH, such as urinary frequency, urgency, and weak urine flow.

It is important to note that a proper diagnosis and treatment plan should be provided by a qualified healthcare professional. If you suspect you have a prostate condition, it is recommended to seek medical advice to receive an accurate evaluation and appropriate care.

Chapter Two

Benefits of Exercise for Prostate Health

The promotion of prostate health is significantly aided by regular exercise, which has many positive effects on general physical fitness. Regular physical exercise has been linked to various advantages for the prostate gland, such as a lower risk of prostate problems, enhanced blood circulation, improved immune function, decreased inflammation, maintenance of a healthy weight, and improved mental health. Men can actively maintain the health of their prostates and lower their chance of acquiring prostate-related illnesses by including exercise into their everyday routines.

The benefits include:

1. Reduced Risk of Prostate Conditions

Engaging in regular physical activity, such as aerobic exercise and strength training, has been associated with a lower risk of developing various prostate conditions, including benign prostatic hyperplasia (BPH) and prostate cancer. Studies have shown that men who lead active lifestyles are less likely to develop these conditions compared to those who are sedentary.

2. Maintenance of Healthy Weight

Exercise plays a crucial role in weight management. Maintaining a healthy weight is important for prostate health as obesity has been linked to an increased risk of developing prostate cancer and BPH. Regular physical activity helps control body weight, reduces excess body fat, and promotes a healthy body composition.

3. Improved Blood Circulation

Exercise promotes better blood circulation throughout the body, including the prostate gland. Improved blood flow helps deliver oxygen and nutrients to the prostate, aiding in its overall health and function. It also helps remove waste products and toxins, keeping the gland in better condition.

4. Enhanced Immune Function

Regular exercise has been shown to strengthen the immune system. A robust immune system is crucial for defending the body against infections, including those that may affect the prostate gland. By strengthening the immune response, exercise may help reduce the risk of prostatitis, a condition characterized by inflammation or infection of the prostate.

5. Decreased Inflammation

Chronic inflammation has been implicated in the development and progression of prostate conditions, including BPH and prostate cancer. Exercise has anti-inflammatory effects on the body, helping to reduce systemic inflammation. By reducing inflammation, exercise may help lower the risk of prostate-related disorders.

6. Better Mental Health

Engaging in regular physical activity has been shown to have positive effects on mental health and well-being. Exercise helps reduce stress, anxiety, and depression, which can indirectly impact prostate health. Stress and negative emotions have been associated with increased inflammation and hormonal imbalances, potentially affecting prostate health. By promoting mental well-being, exercise may indirectly support prostate health.

7. Hormonal Balance

Regular exercise can help promote hormonal balance in the body. Hormonal imbalances, such as elevated levels of estrogen or decreased levels of testosterone, have been associated with an increased risk of prostate conditions, including prostate cancer. Exercise can help regulate hormone levels and contribute to a healthier hormonal profile.

8. Improved Bowel Function

Exercise has been linked to improved bowel function and regularity. A healthy digestive system and regular bowel movements help reduce the risk of constipation and the build-up of toxins in the body. By maintaining a healthy bowel function, exercise may indirectly support prostate health by preventing the accumulation of harmful substances in the prostate gland.

9. Better Sexual Function

Regular physical activity can positively impact sexual function, including erectile function. Erectile dysfunction (ED) is a common concern among men, and it can be associated with various prostate conditions. Exercise improves blood flow, cardiovascular health, and overall vascular function, which are all essential for healthy sexual function. By promoting cardiovascular fitness and circulation, exercise may help reduce the risk of ED and support prostate health.

10. Enhanced Overall Well-being

Exercise contributes to overall well-being and quality of life. It can improve energy levels, sleep quality, and overall vitality. Engaging in regular physical activity can also reduce the risk of developing chronic diseases, such as heart disease, diabetes, and obesity, which are associated with an increased risk of prostate conditions. By promoting general health and well-being, exercise supports prostate health as part of a holistic approach to maintaining overall wellness.

It's important to note that while exercise can have numerous benefits for prostate health, it should be combined with a balanced diet, regular medical check-ups, and a healthy lifestyle overall. As always, it's advisable to consult with a healthcare professional before starting any exercise program or making significant changes to your lifestyle.

Chapter Three

Best Practices for Exercise and Prostate Health

The general health of men depends on maintaining a healthy prostate. Exercise is extremely important for promoting prostate health, in addition to routine check-ups and a balanced diet. Physical activity has been linked to a number of advantages, including increased blood circulation, improved immune function, reduced inflammation, weight control, and improved mental health. Men can actively promote their prostate health and lower their risk of acquiring illnesses related to the prostate by following best practices for exercise.

Consultation with a Healthcare Professional

While exercise typically improves prostate health, it's crucial to remember that individual circumstances and medical conditions might change. In light of this, it is always advisable to seek medical advice before beginning any workout program or altering your lifestyle significantly. A medical expert, such as a primary care doctor or urologist, can offer specialized advice based on your unique medical history, present health condition, and particular needs.

You can address any existing medical issues, prescription drugs, and any particular worries or restrictions you may have with a healthcare expert during a consultation. They can aid in determining how you are feeling generally and offer suggestions that are based on your particular circumstances. This will guarantee that your workout regimen is consistent with your health-related goals and minimizes any potential risk.

Choosing Suitable Exercises

It's important to take into account a number of variables, including personal preferences, fitness level, and any underlying medical concerns, while selecting the right exercises. Regular physical exercise is essential for general health and wellbeing, including prostate health. You may maximize the advantages and reduce the hazards associated with your fitness regimen by choosing exercises that are in line with your capabilities and goals.

Customizing your exercise routine to meet your specific demands is essential, whether it is aerobic exercises, strength training, pelvic floor exercises, or flexibility and balance drills. Selecting appropriate exercises that support prostate health and add to your overall fitness journey can benefit greatly from the advice of a healthcare practitioner or exercise specialist.

Here are some general guidelines to consider when selecting exercises for prostate health:

1. Aerobic Exercises

Include aerobic exercises that elevate your heart rate and promote cardiovascular fitness. Examples include brisk walking, jogging, cycling, swimming, dancing, or using cardio machines like elliptical trainers or rowing machines. Aim for moderate-intensity aerobic activities that you enjoy and can sustain for at least 30 minutes per session.

2. Strength Training

Incorporate strength training exercises to build and maintain muscle strength. This can include using free weights, weight machines, resistance bands, or bodyweight exercises like push-ups, squats, and lunges. Focus on targeting major muscle groups, such as the legs, arms, chest, back, and core. Aim for two to three sessions per week, allowing for recovery time between workouts.

3. Pelvic Floor Exercises

Engage in pelvic floor exercises, also known as Kegel exercises, which specifically target the muscles that support the bladder and prostate. These exercises can help improve urinary control and may benefit individuals with prostate conditions like BPH or post-surgical recovery. Consult with a healthcare professional or a pelvic floor physical therapist to learn the proper technique and recommended routine for pelvic floor exercises.

4. Flexibility and Balance Exercises

Incorporate flexibility and balance exercises to improve overall mobility and stability. Stretching exercises, yoga, tai chi, or Pilates can help enhance flexibility and balance, reducing the risk of falls and improving overall physical function.

5. Low-Impact Exercises

If you have joint problems or conditions that limit high-impact activities, consider low-impact exercises that are gentle on the joints. These can include swimming, water aerobics, stationary biking, or using an elliptical machine. These exercises provide cardiovascular benefits without putting excessive stress on the joints.

6. Mind-Body Exercises

Incorporate mind-body exercises such as yoga or tai chi, which focus on the integration of physical movement, breath control, and mental relaxation. These exercises can help reduce stress, improve flexibility, and promote overall well-being.

7. Considerations for Pre-existing Conditions

If you have pre-existing health conditions, such as arthritis, joint problems, or cardiovascular issues, it's crucial to consult with a healthcare professional or an exercise specialist. They can help tailor an exercise program to your specific needs, considering any limitations or modifications necessary to ensure safety and effectiveness.

Remember to start gradually and listen to your body. It's essential to warm up before exercising and cool down afterward. If you experience any pain, discomfort, or unusual symptoms during or after exercise, consult with a healthcare professional.

Incorporating a variety of exercises into your routine can provide a well-rounded approach to prostate health. Focus on finding activities that you enjoy and that align with your physical capabilities. Regular exercise, tailored to your needs, can contribute to improved prostate health, overall fitness, and well-being.

Frequency, Duration, and Intensity of Exercise

You have to realize that there is no one method that works for everyone when it comes to exercising for prostate health. Based on individual criteria including age, fitness level, general health, and personal goals, the frequency, length, and intensity of exercise might vary greatly. To maximize the advantages and reduce the risks, it is essential to modify your fitness program to fit your unique situation.

The first step is to recognize the value of prostate health and the contribution that exercise makes to preserving it. Prostate cancer and benign prostatic hyperplasia (BPH), two disorders that affect the prostate, have been linked to regular physical exercise. Additionally, it can raise quality of life and general well-being.

It's important to strike the correct balance between exercise intensity, frequency, and duration. To prevent overexertion or injury, it's critical to take into account your present level of fitness and gradually increase your workout schedule. When creating an exercise program that is customized to your unique needs and goals, consulting with a healthcare expert or an exercise specialist can be quite helpful.

You can pick appropriate exercises that support prostate health and add to your overall fitness and well-being by being aware of the significance of individual factors and collaborating closely with healthcare providers.

Here are some general guidelines to consider:

- **Frequency**

Aim for regular exercise sessions throughout the week. The American Heart Association recommends at least 150 minutes of moderate-intensity aerobic activity or 75 minutes of vigorous-intensity aerobic activity per week. This can be achieved through 30 minutes of exercise on most days of the week or by breaking it down into shorter sessions if needed. Additionally, including strength training exercises two to three times a week is beneficial.

- **Duration**

For aerobic exercises, aim for sessions lasting at least 30 minutes. This can be accumulated in shorter bouts of 10-15 minutes throughout the day if needed. The duration of strength training sessions can vary based on the exercises performed and the number of sets and repetitions. Starting with 15-20 minutes of strength training and gradually increasing as tolerated is a good approach.

- **Intensity**

The intensity of aerobic exercise can be measured using the rate of perceived exertion (RPE) scale or by monitoring your heart rate. Moderate-intensity aerobic exercise should make you feel somewhat breathless but still able to carry on a conversation. Vigorous-intensity aerobic exercise will make you breathe harder and make it difficult to carry on a conversation. Strength training exercises should challenge your muscles without causing pain or excessive strain.

- **Gradual Progression**

It's important to start at a comfortable level and gradually increase the frequency, duration, and intensity of exercise over time. This allows your body to adapt and reduces the risk of injury. If you're new to exercise or have any health concerns, consult with a healthcare professional or a certified exercise specialist to determine a suitable starting point and develop a safe and effective progression plan.

Remember, these are general guidelines, and it's important to listen to your body and adjust your exercise routine accordingly. If you have any pre-existing medical conditions or concerns, consult with a healthcare professional to receive personalized recommendations tailored to your individual needs.

Warm-up and Cool-down Routines

All exercise programs, particularly those aimed at promoting prostate health, should include warm-up and cool-down exercises. They support your body's readiness for physical exercise and healing afterward.

Here is a breakdown of warm-up and cool-down exercises:

1. Warm-up

Before starting any exercise session, it's important to warm up your muscles and increase your heart rate gradually. A proper warm-up routine helps prepare your body for the upcoming physical activity and reduces the risk of injury.

Some key elements of a warm-up routine include:

- Light aerobic activity: Begin with a few minutes of low-intensity aerobic exercise, such as brisk walking or gentle cycling. This helps raise your heart rate and increases blood flow to your muscles.

- Dynamic stretching: Perform dynamic stretches that involve active movements through a full range of motion. These stretches help improve flexibility, enhance joint mobility, and activate the muscles you'll be using during your workout. Examples include leg swings, arm circles, or walking lunges.

- Sport-specific movements: Incorporate movements that mimic the activities you'll be performing during your exercise session. For example, if you're planning to jog, include a few minutes of light jogging as part of your warm-up.

The duration of a warm-up routine can vary but typically lasts around 5-10 minutes. Adjust the intensity and duration based on the type and intensity of your planned workout.

2. Cool-down

After completing your exercise session, it's important to gradually bring your heart rate back to its resting state and allow your body to recover. A proper cool-down routine helps reduce muscle soreness, prevent dizziness or lightheadedness, and promote the removal of metabolic waste products.

Here are some elements to include in your cool-down routine:

- Low-intensity aerobic activity: Gradually decrease the intensity of your exercise by transitioning to a lower-intensity activity, such as walking or slow cycling. This helps bring your heart rate down gradually.

- Static stretching: Perform static stretches, holding each stretch for 15-30 seconds, to help improve flexibility and prevent muscle tightness. Focus on stretching the major muscle groups used during your workout.

- Deep breathing and relaxation: Take a few moments to focus on deep breathing and relaxation techniques. This can help reduce tension and promote a sense of calmness and well-being.

Similar to the warm-up, the duration of a cool-down routine is typically around 5-10 minutes, but it can be longer if needed.

By incorporating both warm-up and cool-down routines into your exercise regimen, you can enhance your overall workout experience, reduce the risk of injury, and support your body's recovery process.

Listening To Your Body and Avoiding Overexertion

Listening to your body and avoiding overexertion during exercise is essential for injury prevention and optimal performance. By paying attention to your body's signals, such as pain, fatigue, or discomfort, you can avoid pushing yourself too hard and reduce the risk of injuries.

Overexertion can lead to fatigue, decreased coordination, and compromised form, negatively impacting your exercise performance. It's important to find the right balance between pushing yourself and knowing when to rest and recover.

By respecting your body's limits, you can maintain a safe and effective exercise routine that promotes overall health and well-being.

Let's consider the followings:

1. Paying attention to your body

It's essential to listen to your body's signals during exercise. This means being aware of how you feel physically and emotionally. Pay attention to any discomfort, pain, or unusual sensations you may experience. If you feel any sharp or persistent pain, dizziness, or shortness of breath, it's important to stop exercising and seek medical attention if needed.

2. Avoiding overexertion

Overexertion occurs when you push your body beyond its limits, leading to excessive physical stress and potential harm. It's important to find the right balance between pushing yourself and knowing when to rest. Here are some tips to avoid overexertion:

3. Start gradually

If you're new to exercise or returning after a long break, start with low-intensity activities and gradually increase the duration and intensity over time. This allows your body to adapt and reduces the risk of overexertion.

4. Use the "talk test"

During aerobic activities, such as brisk walking or jogging, you can use the "talk test" to monitor your intensity. If you can carry on a conversation without feeling excessively breathless, you're likely exercising at a moderate intensity. If you're struggling to speak, you may be pushing too hard.

5. Listen to fatigue signals

Fatigue is a natural response to exercise, but excessive fatigue can be a sign of overexertion. If you feel overly tired, weak, or unable to maintain proper form during exercises, it's a signal to take a break and allow your body to recover.

6. Rest and recovery

Rest days are an essential part of any exercise routine. Allow your body time to recover and repair itself between workouts. This helps prevent overuse injuries and supports optimal performance.

By listening to your body's signals, being mindful of your limitations, and avoiding overexertion, you can engage in exercise routines that promote prostate health while minimizing the risk of injury and promoting overall well-being. Remember to consult with a healthcare professional or exercise specialist for personalized guidance based on your individual needs and circumstances.

Staying Consistent with an Exercise Routine

Staying consistent with an exercise routine is key to reaping the benefits of regular physical activity and maintaining prostate health. The importance are as follows:

- **Establishing a Habit**

Consistency helps to establish exercise as a habit in your daily life. By making exercise a regular part of your routine, it becomes easier to stick to and less likely to be skipped or neglected. Set a schedule and dedicate specific times for exercise, just as you would for other important activities.

- **Long-Term Benefits**

Regular exercise provides cumulative benefits for prostate health. Consistency allows your body to adapt and improve over time. It helps to maintain muscle strength, cardiovascular fitness, and overall physical well-being. By staying consistent, you maximize the positive impact on your prostate health and reduce the risk of developing prostate conditions.

- **Motivation and Progress**

Consistency creates a positive feedback loop that fuels motivation and progress. As you stick to your exercise routine, you will likely experience improvements in strength, endurance, and overall fitness.

These positive changes can serve as motivation to keep going and challenge yourself further. Consistent progress can boost confidence and reinforce the importance of maintaining a regular exercise routine.

- **Mental and Emotional Well-being**

Consistency in exercise not only benefits your physical health but also positively impacts your mental and emotional well-being. Regular physical activity has been shown to reduce stress, anxiety, and symptoms of depression. It can boost mood, improve sleep quality, and enhance overall mental resilience. By staying consistent, you can enjoy the mental and emotional rewards that exercise provides.

- **Accountability and Support**

Consistency in exercise can be facilitated by accountability and support systems. Engage in activities that hold you accountable, such as exercising with a partner, joining a fitness class, or tracking your progress. Seek support from friends, family, or online communities to stay motivated and share experiences. Having a support system can make it easier to stay consistent and provide encouragement during challenging times.

When you prioritize consistency in your exercise routine, you can establish a sustainable and beneficial habit that supports prostate health and overall well-being. Remember to consult a healthcare professional or exercise specialist to design a personalized exercise plan that suits your needs and abilities.

Chapter Four

Exercise Tips for Specific Prostate Conditions

When it comes to prostate issues, exercise might be a helpful supplement to your overall care strategy. However, it's crucial to take into account the particular requirements and restrictions related to each prostate condition. Exercise can help with symptoms, promote general health, and enhance treatment outcomes whether you have prostate cancer, prostatitis, or benign prostatic hyperplasia (BPH).

We'll offer exercise ideas in this guide that are specific to each prostate ailment, taking into account personal preferences and recommendations. Always get advice from a competent exercise specialist or your healthcare provider when creating a customized exercise program to meet your goals and limitations.

These include:

Benign Prostatic Hyperplasia (BPH)

For individuals with Benign Prostatic Hyperplasia (BPH), there are exercise modifications that can be beneficial in managing the condition.

- Choose aerobic exercises that are low-impact and gentle on the joints, such as walking, swimming, or cycling and using elliptical machines are excellent options as they provide cardiovascular benefits without putting excessive strain on the prostate.

- Incorporate pelvic floor exercises (Kegel exercises) to strengthen the muscles that support the bladder and prostate.

- Avoid activities that involve heavy lifting, intense straining, or jarring movements that can exacerbate BPH symptoms as they can put pressure on the prostate gland.

- Gradually increase exercise intensity and duration over time to improve overall fitness and manage weight. However, it's crucial to listen to your body and avoid overexertion. If you experience discomfort or a worsening of symptoms, consider reducing the intensity or duration of your exercises and consult with a healthcare professional for guidance.

- Fluid intake is another factor to consider during exercise for BPH. It's crucial to stay adequately hydrated to prevent dehydration and maintain overall health. However, it's recommended to avoid excessive fluid intake just before or during exercise, as it may increase the need for frequent bathroom visits. Finding the right balance in fluid intake can help manage urinary symptoms and discomfort during physical activity.

Prostatitis

When dealing with prostatitis, exercises that encourage blood circulation and lessen inflammation in the pelvic area are crucial for proper management. The following exercises are suggested:

- Engage in low-impact aerobic exercises like walking or stationary cycling to improve blood flow and reduce inflammation. Aim for at least 30 minutes of aerobic exercise most days of the week.

- Practice relaxation techniques, such as yoga or deep breathing exercises, to manage stress and promote relaxation. Certain yoga poses, such as the child's pose, cat-cow, and pigeon pose, may provide relief and promote pelvic relaxation.

- Pelvic Floor Exercises: Pelvic floor exercises, also known as Kegel exercises, can help strengthen the muscles of the pelvic floor and improve urinary control. To perform Kegel exercises, squeeze and hold the muscles you would use to stop the flow of urine. Hold for a few seconds and then release. Repeat this exercise several times throughout the day, gradually increasing the duration of the holds.

- Avoid activities that may exacerbate symptoms, such as high-impact exercises or heavy lifting.

- Consult with a physical therapist who specializes in pelvic floor rehabilitation for specific exercises to help relieve prostatitis symptoms.

Prostate Cancer

During prostate cancer treatment, exercise can play a crucial role in managing side effects, promoting overall well-being, and supporting the treatment process. However, it's important to consult with your healthcare team before starting any exercise program to ensure it is appropriate for your specific situation. Here are some considerations for exercise during prostate cancer treatment:

- Consult with your healthcare team or a certified cancer exercise specialist to develop an individualized exercise plan based on your treatment stage and overall health.

- Fatigue Management: Fatigue is a common side effect of cancer treatment. Adjusting the intensity, duration, and frequency of exercise can help manage fatigue. Start with shorter durations and lower intensities, gradually increasing as tolerated. Listen to your body and rest when needed.

- Incorporate a combination of aerobic exercises (e.g., walking, swimming) and strength training exercises (e.g., resistance training) to maintain cardiovascular fitness and muscle strength. Focus on major muscle groups, such as the arms, legs, back, and core. Start with lighter weights or resistance bands and gradually progress.

- Flexibility and Balance: Include stretching exercises and activities that improve flexibility and balance, such as yoga, tai chi, or Pilates. These exercises can help maintain mobility, reduce muscle tension, and enhance overall physical function.

- Modify exercises based on any treatment-related side effects or physical limitations you may experience.

- Listen to your body and adjust exercise intensity and duration as needed to prevent overexertion and fatigue.

Erectile Dysfunction (ED) Related to Prostate Conditions

Erectile dysfunction (ED) can be a common concern for individuals with prostate conditions, such as benign prostatic hyperplasia (BPH) or prostate cancer. These conditions can affect the prostate gland and its surrounding structures, leading to difficulties in achieving or maintaining an erection.

While the treatment for ED related to prostate conditions may vary depending on the underlying cause and individual circumstances, incorporating certain lifestyle changes and exercises can be helpful. Regular aerobic exercises, such as brisk walking, jogging, or cycling, can improve cardiovascular health and blood flow, which is important for erectile function.

Pelvic floor exercises, also known as Kegel exercises, can strengthen the muscles involved in erectile function and help manage ED symptoms. It is recommended to consult with a healthcare professional or a pelvic floor physical therapist for guidance on specific exercises and treatment options tailored to your condition.

- Engage in aerobic exercises that promote cardiovascular health, such as walking, jogging, or cycling, as they can improve blood flow and overall vascular health.

- Include strength training exercises that target major muscle groups, as they can improve overall fitness and support sexual health.

- Incorporate pelvic floor exercises, such as Kegel exercises, which can help improve blood flow to the pelvic region and strengthen the muscles involved in erectile function.

- Discuss with your healthcare professional about any specific exercises or rehabilitation programs designed to address ED related to prostate conditions.

Post-Prostatectomy Recovery

Post-prostatectomy recovery refers to the period of healing and rehabilitation following a surgical removal of the prostate gland, typically performed to treat prostate cancer. The recovery process is important to regain strength, promote healing, and restore normal function after the procedure.

Below are some key considerations for post-prostatectomy recovery:

- It is crucial to closely follow the post-operative instructions provided by the healthcare team. This may include taking prescribed medications, managing pain, and following dietary guidelines.

- Maintain a healthy and balanced diet to support healing and overall well-being. Adequate nutrition, including lean proteins, fruits, vegetables, whole grains, and healthy fats, can aid in recovery.

- Begin with gentle exercises, such as walking or light stretching, as soon as your healthcare professional gives you the green light after surgery.

- Gradually progress to more challenging activities, under the guidance of a physical therapist or exercise specialist, to regain strength, flexibility, and endurance.

- Focus on strengthening the core muscles, including the pelvic floor muscles, to support overall recovery and urinary control.

- Avoid high-impact exercises or activities that put excessive strain on the surgical area, especially in the early stages of recovery.

- Pelvic Floor Exercises: Pelvic floor exercises, also known as Kegel exercises, are essential for regaining urinary control and restoring pelvic muscle strength. Consult with a healthcare professional or a pelvic floor physical therapist to learn the proper technique and develop a personalized exercise plan.

- Emotional well-being is an important aspect of recovery. Seek support from loved ones, join support groups, or consider counseling to cope with any emotional challenges that may arise during the recovery process.

- Give yourself time to heal and allow your body to recover. Be patient with the recovery process, as it can take several weeks or months to fully regain strength and function.

Remember to always consult with your healthcare professional or an exercise specialist who can provide personalized recommendations based on your specific prostate condition, treatment plan, and overall health. They can help you develop an exercise program that is safe, effective, and tailored to your needs and abilities.

Chapter Five

Additional Lifestyle Factors for Prostate Health

A number of lifestyle choices, in addition to consistent exercise, are essential for preserving prostate health. These lifestyle habits cover a range of daily activities, such as eating right, staying hydrated, managing weight, quitting smoking, managing stress, getting regular checkups, and more. You may support prostate health, lower the risk of prostate disorders, and improve general wellbeing by adopting these extra lifestyle variables into your daily routine.

These lifestyle factors are as follows:

1. Balanced Diet

Adopting a balanced and nutritious diet is crucial for prostate health. This entails including a variety of fruits, vegetables, whole grains, lean proteins (such as fish, poultry, and legumes), and healthy fats (such as avocados, nuts, and olive oil) in your meals. You have to limit the intake of red and processed meats, high-fat dairy products, sugary foods, and processed snacks. Emphasize foods rich in antioxidants, vitamins (especially vitamin D), and minerals like selenium and zinc, as they have been associated with prostate health.

2. Hydration

Staying hydrated is important for overall health, including prostate health. Adequate water intake helps maintain proper urinary function and can reduce the risk of urinary tract infections. Aim to drink at least 8 glasses (64 ounces) of water per day, or adjust based on individual needs and activity levels.

3. Maintain a Healthy Weight

Obesity has been linked to an increased risk of prostate conditions, including prostate cancer and benign prostatic hyperplasia (BPH). Maintain a healthy weight through a combination of regular physical activity and a balanced diet. Losing excess weight, especially around the waistline, can have a positive impact on prostate health.

4. Quit Smoking

Smoking is associated with an increased risk of developing prostate cancer and can worsen the symptoms of prostate conditions. Quitting smoking is one of the best things you can do for your overall health, including prostate health. Seek support from healthcare professionals or smoking cessation programs to help you quit.

5. Limit Alcohol Consumption

Excessive alcohol consumption has been linked to an increased risk of prostate cancer. If you choose to drink alcohol, do so in moderation. The American Cancer Society recommends limiting alcohol intake to no more than 2 drinks per day for men.

6. Stress Management and relaxation techniques

Chronic stress can have negative effects on overall health, including prostate health.

Engage in stress-reducing activities such as exercise, relaxation techniques (e.g., deep breathing, meditation, and yoga), and hobbies, spending time with loved ones, and seeking support when needed. Finding healthy ways to manage stress can help support prostate health.

7. Regular Check-ups and Screenings

Regular visits to a healthcare professional are essential for prostate health. Follow recommended screening guidelines for prostate cancer, including prostate-specific antigen (PSA) blood tests and digital rectal exams. Early detection can significantly improve treatment outcomes.

8. Sleep Quality

Adequate sleep is crucial for overall health and well-being, including prostate health. Aim for 7-9 hours of quality sleep per night. Develop good sleep hygiene habits, such as maintaining a regular sleep schedule, creating a comfortable sleep environment, and practicing relaxation techniques before bed.

9. Limit Exposure to Environmental Toxins

Minimize exposure to environmental toxins and chemicals that may affect prostate health. For example, use protective equipment when working with hazardous substances, avoid prolonged exposure to pesticides and herbicides, and choose organic or locally sourced food options when possible.

10. Open Communication and Education

Stay informed about prostate health and conditions. Be proactive in discussing any concerns or symptoms with your healthcare provider.

Educate yourself about the signs and symptoms of prostate conditions and the importance of regular check-ups.

Remember, it is important to consult with a healthcare professional for personalized advice and guidance on maintaining prostate health. They can provide specific recommendations based on your individual needs, medical history, and risk factors.

Chapter Six

Precautions and Considerations

Maintaining prostate health and controlling diseases related to the prostate need taking care and taking certain aspects into account. Understanding the essential precautions will help you make informed decisions and take proactive measures toward achieving optimal prostate health, whether you have been diagnosed with a prostate disease or want to prevent future issues.

The important precautions and considerations to bear in mind to support prostate health and general wellbeing, from lifestyle choices to medical advice, will be listed. You may take charge of your prostate health and support a greater quality of life by adhering to these suggestions and getting individualized guidance from healthcare experts.

1. Follow Medical Advice

It is crucial to follow the advice and treatment plan prescribed by your healthcare provider. They will provide specific guidance based on your prostate condition, such as prostatitis, benign prostatic hyperplasia (BPH), or prostate cancer. Adhering to the recommended treatments and lifestyle modifications is important for managing and improving your condition.

2. Limit Alcohol Consumption

While moderate alcohol consumption may be acceptable for some individuals, it's generally advisable to limit or avoid alcohol if you have a prostate condition. Alcohol can exacerbate symptoms, such as urinary problems, inflammation, or irritation in the prostate gland. Consult with your healthcare provider to determine if alcohol consumption is safe in your specific case.

3. Hydration

Staying properly hydrated is important for prostate health. Drinking an adequate amount of water can help flush out toxins and maintain urinary tract health. Ensure you maintain good hydration habits, especially if you experience urinary symptoms related to your prostate condition.

4. Dietary Considerations

Pay attention to your diet and make choices that support prostate health. Consider incorporating foods that are rich in antioxidants, such as fruits, vegetables, and whole grains. Some studies suggest that a diet low in red meat and high in plant-based proteins may be beneficial for prostate health. Consult with a healthcare provider or a registered dietitian for personalized dietary recommendations.

5. Regular Follow-ups and Screenings

If you have a prostate condition or a history of prostate issues, it's important to schedule regular follow-up appointments and screenings with your healthcare provider. Regular check-ups can help monitor your condition, detect any changes or progression, and ensure timely intervention if needed.

6. Stress Management

Chronic stress can potentially worsen symptoms related to prostate conditions. Explore stress management techniques such as exercise, meditation, deep breathing, or engaging in activities you enjoy. Managing stress levels can positively impact your overall well-being, including prostate health.

7. Exercise Regularly

Regular physical activity can have positive effects on prostate health. Engaging in moderate exercise, such as brisk walking, jogging, or cycling, can help improve circulation, manage weight, and reduce the risk of certain prostate conditions. However, consult with your healthcare provider before starting any exercise regimen to ensure it is appropriate for your condition.

8. Maintain a Healthy Weight

Excess weight, especially around the waistline, can increase the risk of prostate problems and complications. Aim to maintain a healthy weight through a balanced diet and regular exercise, as weight management can positively impact prostate health.

9. Quit Smoking

If you smoke, consider quitting. Smoking has been linked to an increased risk of prostate cancer and can worsen symptoms in individuals with prostate conditions. Seek support from healthcare professionals or smoking cessation programs to quit smoking and improve your overall health.

10. Educate Yourself

Take the time to educate yourself about your specific prostate condition. Understand the symptoms, treatment options, and potential complications associated with your condition. This knowledge can help you make informed decisions and actively participate in your healthcare.

11. Seek Support

Dealing with a prostate condition can be emotionally challenging. Consider seeking support from friends, family, or support groups. Connecting with others who have similar experiences can provide valuable insight, advice, and emotional support.

12. Recognizing Warning Signs and Seeking Medical Attention

Early detection and timely medical attention play a crucial role in managing prostate health. It's important to be aware of the warning signs associated with prostate conditions and to seek medical attention promptly if any symptoms arise. By recognizing these signs and taking appropriate action, you can ensure that potential issues are addressed promptly and effectively.

If you experience any symptoms associated with prostate conditions, such as frequent urination, difficulty starting or stopping urination, weak urine flow, blood in urine or semen, pain or discomfort in the pelvic area, or erectile dysfunction, it's essential to take them seriously. While some symptoms may be benign, they can also indicate underlying prostate issues, including prostatitis, benign prostatic hyperplasia (BPH), or prostate cancer. Ignoring or dismissing these symptoms can lead to delayed diagnosis and treatment.

Consulting with a healthcare professional, such as a urologist or primary care physician, is crucial if you notice warning signs or have concerns about your prostate health. Schedule an appointment to discuss your symptoms, medical history, and any relevant information. The healthcare professional will conduct a thorough evaluation and may recommend further tests or examinations to accurately diagnose your condition.

Depending on your age, medical history, and risk factors, your healthcare provider may recommend prostate screenings, such as a prostate-specific antigen (PSA) blood test or a digital rectal examination (DRE). These screenings can help detect potential abnormalities or signs of prostate conditions. Regular screenings may be advised for individuals at higher risk or those with a history of prostate problems. It's important to follow your healthcare provider's recommendations regarding screening frequency and any additional diagnostic tests that may be necessary.

Effective communication with your healthcare provider is essential during the evaluation and treatment process. Be open and honest about your symptoms, medical history, lifestyle choices, and any relevant information that can assist in the diagnosis. This will help your healthcare provider make an accurate assessment and provide appropriate care and guidance tailored to your specific needs.

Remember, early detection and timely medical attention can significantly improve outcomes for prostate conditions. If you notice warning signs or have any concerns, don't hesitate to seek medical advice. Your healthcare provider is the best resource to evaluate your symptoms, provide an accurate diagnosis, and guide you through the appropriate steps for managing your prostate health.

Conclusion

Regular exercise plays a crucial role in maintaining prostate health and overall well-being. Engaging in physical activity offers numerous benefits that can positively impact the prostate and reduce the risk of prostate-related conditions. Exercise promotes better blood circulation and oxygen delivery to the prostate, supporting its health and function. It also helps regulate hormone levels, reduce inflammation, and boost immune function, all of which contribute to a healthy prostate. Additionally, exercise aids in weight management, which is important as excess weight, especially around the waistline, is associated with a higher risk of prostate issues. By incorporating regular exercise into your routine, you can enhance prostate health and reduce the likelihood of developing prostate conditions.

To reap the benefits of exercise for prostate health, aim for a combination of cardiovascular activities and strength training exercises. Cardiovascular exercises, such as brisk walking, jogging, cycling, or swimming, help improve circulation and strengthen the heart. Strength training exercises, such as weightlifting or resistance training, help build muscle mass and improve overall strength. It's important to start gradually, especially if you're new to exercise or have any underlying health conditions. Consult with a healthcare professional or a qualified fitness expert to develop a personalized exercise plan that suits your abilities and goals. Remember to listen to your body, stay hydrated, and warm up before exercising to prevent injury.

Incorporating regular exercise into your lifestyle not only supports prostate health but also provides overall health benefits. It can help manage weight, reduce the risk of chronic diseases, improve mood, and boost energy levels. By making exercise a priority, you are taking proactive steps towards maintaining optimal prostate health and promoting your overall well-being.

Adopting an active lifestyle is one of the best investments you can make for your overall well-being. Regular physical activity offers a multitude of benefits that extend beyond just physical health. It has a profound impact on your mental, emotional, and social well-being, leading to a higher quality of life. Here's some encouragement to embrace an active lifestyle:

Engaging in regular exercise helps strengthen your muscles, bones, and cardiovascular system. It can help manage weight, reduce the risk of chronic diseases such as heart disease, diabetes, and certain types of cancer, and improve overall physical fitness. Regular physical activity also boosts your energy levels, enhances flexibility and balance, and promotes better sleep patterns. By adopting an active lifestyle, you are investing in a healthier, stronger, and more resilient body.

Physical activity has a positive impact on your mental and emotional health. Exercise releases endorphins, also known as "feel-good" hormones, which can elevate your mood, reduce stress, anxiety, and symptoms of depression, and improve cognitive function. It provides an outlet for managing and coping with everyday stressors, enhances self-esteem, and boosts overall mental well-being. By staying active, you are nurturing your mind and emotions, leading to increased happiness and a more positive outlook on life.

Participating in physical activities often opens doors to new social connections and a sense of community. Whether it's joining a sports team, participating in group fitness classes, or simply going for a walk with friends or family, exercise can foster social interactions and create meaningful relationships. Being part of a community that shares common interests and goals provides a sense of belonging and support, which is vital for overall well-being. By embracing an active lifestyle, you can broaden your social circles and enjoy the benefits of shared experiences and camaraderie.

Embracing an active lifestyle is not about becoming an elite athlete or adhering to a strict exercise regimen. It's about finding activities you enjoy and incorporating movement into your daily routine. Whether it's walking, dancing, swimming, cycling, hiking, or practicing yoga, the key is to engage in activities that bring you joy and keep you consistently active.

Start small and gradually increase the duration and intensity of your activities. Set realistic goals and celebrate your progress along the way. Remember, every step counts, and even small bursts of activity throughout the day can have a positive impact on your overall well-being.

So, let this be an encouragement to prioritize your health and happiness by embracing an active lifestyle. Take the first step today and experience the transformative power of regular physical activity for your body, mind, and soul. Your well-being deserves it!

References

Hackshaw-McGeagh, L. E., Perry, R. E., Leach, V. A., Qandil, S., Jeffreys, M., Martin, R. M., & Lane, J. A. (2016). A systematic review of dietary, nutritional, and physical activity interventions for the prevention of prostate cancer progression and mortality. Cancer Causes & Control, 27(6), 745-757.

https://atlanticurologyclinics.com/conditions/prostatitis-infection-of-the-prostate/

https://medika.life/the-prostate-gland/

https://www.cancer.gov/about-cancer/causes-prevention/risk/alcohol/alcohol-fact-sheet

https://www.cancer.org/cancer/cancer-causes/diet-physical-activity/alcohol-use-and-cancer.html

https://www.cdc.gov/cancer/prostate/basic_info/alcohol-use.htm

https://www.mayoclinic.org/diseases-conditions/prostate-cancer/expert-answers/prostate-cancer/faq-20058346

https://www.pcf.org/c/prostate-cancer-risk-factors/

https://www.pcfa.org.au/awareness/general-information/understanding-prostate-cancer/what-is-the-prostate/

Kenfield, S. A., Stampfer, M. J., Giovannucci, E., & Chan, J. M. (2011). Physical activity and survival after prostate cancer diagnosis in the health professionals follow-up study. Journal of Clinical Oncology, 29(6), 726-732.

Leitzmann, M. F., & Rohrmann, S. (2012). Risk factors for the onset of prostatic cancer: Age, location, and behavioral correlates. Clinical Epidemiology, 4(Suppl 1), 1-11.

Parsons, J. K., Newman, V. A., Mohler, J. L., Pierce, J. P., Flatt, S. W., Marshall, J., ... & Hamilton, A. S. (2015). Physical activity, sitting time, and incident prostate cancer risk: Results from the CaPSURE prostate cancer cohort. Cancer Causes & Control, 26(11), 1615-1621.